LUPUS DIET FOR THE NEWLY DIAGNOSED

Recipes to ease Inflammation, Treat Flares, and manage Lupus into Remission with meal plans

Copyright ©2023.

`

TABLE OF CONTENTS

FOREWORD

My name is Sarah and I'm a twenty-five year old college student. I had been feeling really tired and run down for months, and it had started to interfere with my ability to study and focus. I went to the doctor and they ran some tests, and after a few weeks they gave me the diagnosis: I had lupus.

At first, I was devastated. I had heard of lupus before, but I didn't really know much about it. I was afraid of what it would do to me, and I felt like my life was over.

But then I started doing some research. I read about how lupus can be managed with diet and exercise, and I realized that I had some control over my condition. I decided to take control, and I started looking for recipes that were healthy and would help me manage my lupus.

I was amazed at how many recipes I found. I was able to find recipes for breakfast, lunch, dinner, snacks, and desserts that were all healthy and free of ingredients that might trigger a lupus flare-up. I was so excited that I decided to compile all of the recipes into a book.

I worked on the book for months, and finally it was finished. I called it "The Lupus Cookbook." It contained all of the recipes I had gathered, as well as some advice on how to manage lupus with diet and exercise.

Since then, my book has been helping people with lupus all over the world. For me, it was an incredible journey of self-discovery and empowerment. I'm proud to say that I'm living a healthy life with lupus, and I owe it all to the recipes I found and the book I put together.

INTRODUCTION TO LUPUS

Welcome to your journey of managing lupus through diet! This cookbook is designed to help you understand what to eat and what to avoid as you explore the world of lupus and nutrition.

Living with lupus can be incredibly challenging. But, with the right diet, you can give yourself the best chance for managing your symptoms and managing your overall health.

This cookbook was written by a lupus patient and nutritionist who understands the importance of nutrition in managing lupus. In this cookbook, you will learn about the foods that can help you manage lupus symptoms and how to create delicious meals that are both nutritious and enjoyable.

With this cookbook, you will have the knowledge and tools you need to make positive changes in your diet as you navigate living with lupus. So, let's get started!

Lupus is associated with multisystemic inflammation resulting from abnormal immunological function. Patients experience periodic flares of varying severity or instances in which no observable signs or symptoms are present. **The four main types of lupus are:**

- Neonatal And Pediatric Lupus Erythematosus (NLE)
- Discoid Lupus Erythematosus (DLE)
- Drug-Induced Lupus (DIL)
- Systemic Lupus Erythematosus (SLE)

DEFINITION OF LUPUS

Systemic lupus erythematosus (SLE), which is simply known as lupus, is an autoimmune disease in which the immune system of the body erroneously onslaughts tissues in various parts of the body which are healthy It may show only single organ sign or multiple system sign at the onset. It can affect the brain, skin, joints and other parts of the body. It is an autoimmune problem that has a wide-ranging clinical presentation, encircling various parts of the body.

Varieties of lupus skin reactions

1. **Acute cutaneous lupus (also called as the butterfly lupus rash or malar rash).**

2. **The subacute cutaneous lupus**: There are two types:

(a) the first one is very sensitive to exposure to the sun and depicts red coloured pimples as the skin eruptions development begins. (b) The second variety begins as flat lesions and get larger as they enlarge to the exterior.

3. **Chronic cutaneous lupus (also called discoid lupus erythematosus—DLE):** these skin eruptions are found in a very few of SLE patients.

The disease SLE can attack people of all ages, races and both males and females, but it has been observed that more than 90% of new patients having SLE are women in their conceiving years. The prevalence of SLE, which has been reported recently, is 20–150 per 100,000. Data from metropolitan areas in the United States stipulated the prevalence to be 104–170 per 100,000 women. The lowest incidence rates are observed in Caucasian populations

Classification

Up to now, it has been divided into two parts:

- The discoid lupus
- The disseminated lupus.

CRITERION DEFINITION

1. **Malar rash Fixed erythema**, flat or raised, over the malar eminences, tending to spare the nasolabial folds

2. **Discoid rash Erythematous** raised patches with adherent keratotic scaling and follicular plugging; atrophic scarring may occur in older lesions

Symptoms

Lupus facial rash

No two cases of lupus are exactly alike. Signs and symptoms may come on suddenly or develop slowly, may be mild or severe, and may be temporary or permanent. Most people with lupus have mild disease characterized by episodes — called flares — when signs and symptoms get worse for a while, then improve or even disappear completely for a time.

The signs and symptoms of lupus that you experience will depend on which body systems are affected by the disease. The most common signs and symptoms include:

- Fatigue
- Fever
- Joint pain, stiffness and swelling

- Butterfly-shaped rash on the face that covers the cheeks and bridge of the nose or rashes elsewhere on the body
- Skin lesions that appear or worsen with sun exposure
- Fingers and toes that turn white or blue when exposed to cold or during stressful periods
- Shortness of breath
- Chest pain
- Dry eyes
- Headaches, confusion and memory loss

CAUSES

As an autoimmune disease, lupus occurs when your immune system attacks healthy tissue in your body. It's likely that lupus results from a combination of your genetics and your environment.

It appears that people with an inherited predisposition for lupus may develop the disease when they come into contact with something in the environment that can trigger lupus. The cause of lupus in most cases, however, is unknown. Some potential triggers include:

- **Sunlight.** Exposure to the sun may bring on lupus skin lesions or trigger an internal response in susceptible people.
- **Infections**. Having an infection can initiate lupus or cause a relapse in some people.
- **Medications**. Lupus can be triggered by certain types of blood pressure medications, anti-seizure medications and antibiotics. People who have drug-induced lupus usually get better when they stop taking the medication. Rarely, symptoms may persist even after the drug is stopped.

Risk factors

Factors that may increase your risk of lupus include:

- Your sex. Lupus is more common in women.
- Age. Although lupus affects people of all ages, it's most often diagnosed between the ages of 15 and 45.
- Race. Lupus is more common in African Americans, Hispanics and Asian Americans.

LUPUS AIP MEAL PLAN

Meal prep option: you can make these recipes ahead of time to save time.

Day 1

- **Breakfast:** Classic AIP Breakfast Hash Template
- **Lunch:** Canned Tuna Pasta (double-batch)
- **Dinner:** Cozy Instant Pot Chili

Day 2

- **Breakfast:** Salmon Cakes over Mixed Greens with Olive Oil and Lemon Juice (double-batch)
- **Lunch:** Canned Tuna Pasta (leftovers)
- **Dinner:** Meatballs over Spaghetti Squash with Pesto

Day 3

- **Breakfast:** Classic AIP Breakfast Hash Template (leftovers)
- **Lunch:** Cozy No-tomato Chili (leftovers)

- **Dinner:** One-pan Chicken and Veggies with Bacon

Day 4

- **Breakfast:** Salmon Cakes over Mixed Greens with Olive Oil and Lemon Juice (leftovers)
- **Lunch:** One-pan Chicken and Veggies with Bacon (leftovers)
- **Dinner:** Cozy No-tomato Chili (leftovers)

Day 5

- **Breakfast:** Classic AIP Breakfast Hash Template (leftovers)
- **Lunch:** Tropical Chicken Salad
- **Dinner:** Picadillo with Plantain Rice

Day 6

- **Breakfast:** Unsweetened Coconut Yogurt with Blueberries and Cinnamon or any leftovers from the week
- **Lunch:** Meatballs over Spaghetti Squash with Pesto (leftovers)

- **Dinner:** Orange Chicken and Broccoli Rice

Day 7

- **Breakfast:** Tigernut Waffles with Strawberries and Cinnamon
- **Lunch:** Orange Chicken and Broccoli Rice (leftovers)
- **Dinner:** Picadillo with Plantain Rice (leftovers)

LUPUS DIET RECIPES

IMMUNE BOOSTING GREEN SMOOTHIE

INGREDIENTS

- Kale Organic*, enough to fill your blender!
- Spinach Organic*, 1-2 cups
- Ginger Root fresh, grated (Organic*)
- Turmeric Root fresh, grated (Organic*)
- 3 Tbsp Flax Seeds or Chia Seeds whole unground
- Walnuts
- Psyllium Husk Powder
- ½ Large Lemon Juiced
- Fruit Of Choice

We use: For 1 large blender-full 1 banana, ⅓ cup organic mango, organic 1/2 apple, a handful of organic blueberries and 1-2 organic strawberries

INSTRUCTIONS

1. Fill blender with kale and spinach (or greens of choice) until ¾ full, pressed down- NOT loose and airy!
2. Add fruit, ginger and turmeric root, psyllium husk powder, and nuts and seeds to the top ¼ of blender
3. Fill with clean drinking water until water level is just above the greens
4. Finally, add the juice of 1 fresh lemon (or half of a large lemon) into the blender! Add extra lemon if desired- it really helps cut down on the "grassy" taste of the greens and allows the fruit to pop!
5. Blend well- and enjoy!

MUSHROOM AND CANNELLINI BEAN SOUP

INGREDIENTS

- 20 g dried mushrooms
- 2 tbsp olive oil
- 1 large red onion, diced
- 2 garlic cloves, crushed

- 2 tbsp fresh thyme
- 100 g fresh Shitake mushrooms, sliced
- 300 g chestnut mushrooms, sliced
- 700 ml vegetable stock
- 400 g can cannellini beans, drained
- seasoning to taste

Optional garnishes

- 1 tbsp pine nuts, toasted
- 1 dsp Extra virgin olive oil
- a few drops of truffle oil
- fresh thyme leaves

INSTRUCTIONS

1. Soak the dried mushrooms in 150ml of warm water for at least 45minutes. Drain the dried mushrooms reserving the liquid.
2. Heat the oil in a large saucepan on a medium heat. Sauté the redonion for five minutes. Add the garlic and thyme. Cook for oneminute, then add the sliced fresh mushrooms.
3. Cook the mushrooms until they are starting to turn golden. Add thedrained (rehydrated)

mushrooms and gently cook for a further sevenminutes.

4. Add the stock and the reserved, strained mushroom liquid (be carefulnot to add any granular bits, sometimes dried mushrooms leave whenthey are refreshed in water). Simmer gently for 10 minutes.

5. Add the drained cannellini beans and season to taste (be careful withsalt if you are using a stock cube and not fresh stock as this will oftenhave added salt). Cook for 10 minutes, partially covered.

6. Blend the soup until smooth. Check the seasoning. Return to thesaucepan and simmer until ready to serve.

7. Toast the pine kernels in a dry frying pan until golden. Garnish the soup with the pine nuts and a drizzle of olive oil (or truffle oil as a treat).

GRAIN FREE BERRY CRISP (AIP)

INGREDIENTS

Fruit Bottom

- 7-8 cups mixed berries whole (can be fresh or frozen)
- 1 Tbsp lemon juice
- 3/4 tsp cinnamon

Topping

- 1 cups cassava flour or arrowroot flour
- 1/2 cup coconut flour
- 1 1/2 cups unsweetened shredded coconut
- 3/4 cup coconut sugar
- 1/2 tsp Celtic sea salt
- 3/4 cup refined coconut oil (melted) or substitute palm shortening

INSTRUCTIONS

Fruit Bottom

1. Mix fruit, lemon juice, and cinnamon. Dump into greased 9 x 13 pan. Should cover

bottom of pan entirely with a layer of fruit about 1 1/2 inches thick.

Topping

1. Combine all ingredients. Stir with fork if using melted coconut oil or use pastry blender for palm shortening. Mix well until combined.
2. Pour topping over fruit bottom and spread evenly. Bake uncovered at 350 degrees Fahrenheit for 30-35 minutes or until golden brown on top.

TOMATO AND COCONUT SOUP

INGREDIENTS

Faux Parmesan Cheese:

- 1 cup raw cashews
- ¼ cup nutritional yeast
- ½ tsp garlic powder
- ¾ tsp kosher salt

Soup:

- 2 Tbsp extra-virgin olive oil

- 1 small yellow onion, diced
- 2 cloves garlic, sliced
- 1 (1-inch) piece ginger, peeled and thinly sliced
- Kosher salt, to taste
- ½ tsp red pepper flakes
- 1 (15-oz) can crushed San Marzano tomatoes
- ¾ cup unsweetened full-fat coconut milk
- Freshly ground black pepper, to taste
- ¼ cup Faux Parmesan Cheese
- 1 Tbsp finely chopped cilantro

INSTRUCTIONS

Faux Parmesan Cheese:

1. Place all ingredients in a blender or food processor. Pulse 10 times or until mixture has consistency of fine crumbs and resembles grated Parmesan cheese. Refrigerate in an airtight container up to 3 weeks. (Makes about 1¼ cups.)

Soup:

1. In a medium saucepan over medium, heat oil until shimmering. Add onion, garlic, ginger and a pinch of salt. Cook 5 minutes or until vegetables are aromatic and soft. Add red pepper flakes; cook, stirring constantly, 30 seconds. Add tomatoes, coconut milk, and a pinch of salt and pepper; bring to a simmer. Cover; cook, stirring occasionally, 15 minutes.

2. Remove from heat. Transfer soup to a blender or food processor. Add Faux Parmesan Cheese; process until smooth. Serve topped with cilantro.

PLANT-BASED CAULIFLOWER QUESADILLA

INGREDIENTS

- 2 Cali'Flour Foods Plant-Based Crust of Choice
- 1/2 cup refried beans
- 1 fresh cut tomato, thinly sliced
- 1/2 cup fresh corn
- 1/4 cup fresh olives

- 1/2 vegan shredded, meltable cheese
- dash of salt and pepper
- handful of fresh cilantro, roughly chopped
- half an avocado, chopped

INSTRUCTIONS

1. Preheat oven to 400F and grab your vented pan to cook your crust on.
2. Remove your crusts from the package and cook one as instructed on the package. Once cooked, remove from the oven and cut in the half. To one half, begin adding all your favourite toppings. For ours, we added refried beans, corn, tomato, olives and vegan cheese. Place the other half of the crust onto the crust with the toppings and cook in the oven at 400F for 7-8 minutes or until perfectly melty and warm.
3. Carefully remove from the oven and enjoy with fresh cilantro, a light dash of lime, salsa and fresh avocado!

HEALTHY VEGAN BLUEBERRY MUFFINS WITH ALMOND MEAL

INGREDIENTS

Dry Ingredients

- 1 cup almond meal
- ¾ cup gluten free all purpose flour
- ½ cup rolled oats
- ½ lemon, zest only
- 1 teaspoon baking soda
- ½ teaspoon salt
- ½ teaspoon cinnamon

Wet Ingredients

- 1 cup unsweetened almond milk, vanilla is nice here
- 1 small ripe banana, mashed
- ¼ cup ground flax
- ¼ cup extra virgin olive oil
- ¼ cup maple syrup
- 2 tablespoons cane sugar
- 1 tablespoon freshly squeezed lemon juice
- 1 teaspoon pure vanilla extract

- 1 cup blueberries, fresh or frozen

INSTRUCTIONS

1. Preheat oven to 375°F (190°C) and line a muffin tin with paper or silicone muffin liners.
2. In a medium bowl, whisk together the flax and ¼ cup hot water, set aside.
3. In a large mixing bowl, whisk together the almond meal, flour, oats, lemon zest, baking soda, salt and cinnamon.
4. In the medium bowl with the gelled flax, add almond milk, mashed banana, olive oil, maple syrup, sugar, lemon juice and vanilla and mix well.
5. Add wet to dry ingredients and stir until well combined. Gently fold in blueberries.
6. Portion out batter into muffin pan using a ¼ cup measure. Bake for 23-25 minutes until tops are golden brown and a toothpick inserted into centre comes out clean.
7. Let muffins cool in the pan for at least 10 minutes before turning out onto cooling rack to cool fully. The muffins will firm up as they cool.

KETO LOW CARB CREAMY TUSCAN CHICKEN

INGREDIENTS

- 6 chicken thighs, or 4 chicken breasts
- salt
- 1 tbsp olive oil
- 1/2 cup red onion , finely diced
- 3 cloves garlic , minced
- Tuscan Chicken Cream Sauce
- ½ cup sun dried tomatoes , chopped
- 2 cups baby spinach
- 1 cup heavy cream
- 1 tsp ground black pepper
- 1 tsp dijon mustard
- 1/2 cup Pecorino Romano cheese , or Parmesan cheese
- 1/2 cup white Cheddar cheese , grated

INSTRUCTIONS

1. Season the chicken on both sides with a little salt and let it sit for 15 minutes.
2. Add the olive oil to a large non stick, or cast iron skillet, over a medium heat.

3. Cook chicken thighs skin side down (if using thighs) for about 12-15 minutes to crisp up the skin, keep it on a medium-low heat so it does not burn.

4. If using chicken breasts brown it works best if you cut large pieces in half lengthways, cook on each side for about 6 minutes per side to brown.

5. Turn the chicken and continue cooking over a medium-low heat for a further 15 minutes or until fully cooked, then remove from the skillet.

6. Add the red onion and garlic to the same skillet and cook until translucent over a medium low heat for three to five minutes until translucent.

7. Add the chopped sun dried tomatoes, spinach, and stir for 30 seconds.

8. Add the heavy cream, black pepper, and bring it to a boil then add the Dijon mustard, cheeses, and simmer over a medium heat until the sauce has thickened. Taste the sauce and season more if needed.

9. Add the chicken back the pan and coat in the sauce and reheat gently if needed.

YUMMY BREADED BAKED CHICKEN

INGREDIENTS

- 2 c Andy's yellow fish breading
- 1 tbs garlic powder
- 1 tsp Himalayan pink salt
- 1 c Shredded Parmesan asiago romano cheese
- 1 c Helmans mayo
- 1 package boneless skinless chicken tenders

INSTRUCTIONS

1. Mix together breading, cheese, garlic, salt. Set aside
2. Tenderize chicken breasts
3. Roll in mayo
4. Toss in breading
5. Place in an oven safe pan and bake for 45 minutes at 400 degre

MEDITERRANEAN LAMB MEATBALLS WITH PALEO TZATZIKI

INGREDIENTS

For Meatballs:

- 1 lb. ground lamb
- 1 cup almond flour
- 1 large egg
- 2 t minced garlic
- 2 T fresh mint, finely chopped
- 2 T lemon zest
- 1 t dried oregano
- 1 t cumin
- 1/4 t onion powder
- 1/4 t ground black pepper
- 1/4 t sea salt
- 2 T avocado oil for cooking

For Paleo Tzatziki:

- 1 cup cashews, soaked in 2 cups water for 6-8 hours
- 1/2 cup unsweetened almond milk

- 1/3 cup chopped cucumber
- 1/4 t dried dill
- 1/2 t minced garlic
- 1/4 t sea salt

INSTRUCTIONS

1. To Make the Meatballs: Combine the meatball ingredients in a medium mixing bowl and use your hands to thoroughly combine. Form the mixture into small balls (about the size of golf balls) and set aside.
2. Heat the avocado oil in a skillet over medium-high heat for 3 minutes. Add six meatballs into the pan and cook for 10 minutes, rotating the meatballs every 2 minutes.
3. When finished, remove the first batch of meatballs from the skillet and repeat with the remaining meatballs.
4. When ready, return all the meatballs back to to the pan and reduce the heat to medium-low. Cover and cook for 10 minutes, or until the meatballs are fully cooked through.
5. To Make the Paleo Tzatziki: In the meantime, combine the ingredients for the

tzatziki in a food processor. Blend until smooth for about 1 minute.

6. When meatballs are ready, serve them hot over a bed of greens and a drizzle the tzatziki on top.

GLUTEN FREE BURGERS

INGREDIENTS

- 1 Lb Ground Beef
- 1/2 Tbsp Worcestershire Sauce
- 1/2 Tbsp Parsley Flakes, Or Fresh Parsley
- 1/2 Tsp Garlic Salt
- 1/2 Tsp Onion Powder
- Romaine Lettuce
- Tomatoes
- Onions
- Swiss Cheese

INSTRUCTIONS

1. In a large bowl, mix together the ground beef, sauce and spices. Note here that you can use any of your favorite hamburger seasonings.

2. Next form patties, this made 4 patties for us. Lastly grill these or cook on medium heat in the skillet. These should cook until well done in the middle or your preference. Normally ours take about 10 minutes on the grill.
3. Once they are done add a layer of cheese and then place the patty in between a few pieces of cut lettuce and pile high with your favorite toppings. Enjoy!

BACON CHEESEBURGER CASSEROLE {PALEO, NO ADDED SUGAR}

INGREDIENTS

cheese sauce:

- 1 1/2 cups cashews no need to soak
- 1/4 cup fresh lemon juice about 2 lemons
- 1/2 cup water
- 1/4 cup olive oil or avocado oil
- 2 tsp garlic powder
- 1 tsp sea salt
- 3 Tbsp nutritional yeast
- remaining ingredients:
- 1 medium yellow onion chopped
- 1 medium red bell pepper diced
- 8 oz mushrooms roughly chopped
- 3 cloves garlic minced
- 1 package (8oz) Jones Dairy Farm No Sugar Hickory Smoked Bacon
- 1 1/2 lbs grass fed ground beef
- Sea salt and black pepper
- 1/2 tsp paprika

- 1/2 tsp onion powder
- Sugar-free ketchup homemade or store bought
- Sliced dill pickles
- Anything else you'd like on your cheeseburger! Jalapeños; avocado sliced red onion, etc.

INSTRUCTIONS

for the cheese sauce:

1. Place all ingredients in a high-speed blender or food processor. I used my NutriBullet for this and it was fast and easy. Blend on high speed until smooth and creamy, set aside.

for the casserole:

1. Preheat your oven to 375 degrees. Heat a large skillet over medium high heat and cook the bacon, in batches if necessary, until crisp. Drain on paper towels and set aside. Reserve 2 Tbsp of the bacon fat.
2. Lower the heat to medium and add the onion, peppers, and mushrooms. Cook for 2-3 minutes until softened, then add the garlic,

stir, and cook another and sprinkle the mixture with sea salt and pepper. Continue to cook 2 more minutes.

3. Push the veggies to one side of the skillet and add the ground beef to the other. Sprinkle with sea salt, pepper, paprika, and onion powder. Cook, using a spatula to break up lumps as it browns. Mix the beef with the veggies and continue to cook until the beef is fully browned, then remove from heat.

4. To assemble, transfer the beef mixture to a 9 x 13 glass casserole dish, then layer with the cheese mixture. Gently stir to combine the two layers, then crumble the cooked bacon over the top. Bake in the preheated oven for 10-15 minutes or until heated through and bubbly.

5. To serve, top the casserole with sliced pickles, ketchup, and any other desired toppings. Store leftovers covered in the refrigerator for up to 3 days. Enjoy!

GINGER & TURMERIC CARROT SOUP

INGREDIENTS

- 1 tablespoon olive oil
- 1 leek , cleaned and sliced
- 1 cup chopped fennel (1 small head)
- 3 cups chopped carrots
- 1 cup chopped butternut squash (or more carrots)
- 2 garlic cloves , minced
- 1 tablespoon grated ginger (about 2" piece)
- 1 tablespoon turmeric powder
- Salt & pepper to taste
- 3 cups low sodium vegetable broth
- 1 (14.5 oz) can lite coconut milk

INSTRUCTIONS

1. Heat the olive oil in a large dutch oven or saucepan. Add the fennel, leeks, carrots, and squash. Saute for 3 - 5 minutes until the veggies start to soften. Add the garlic, ginger, turmeric, salt, and pepper, and saute for a few more minutes.

2. Add the broth and coconut milk. Bring the mixture to a boil, cover and simmer for 20 minutes.

3. Once the soup is cooked, add it to a blender and blend until creamy. You could also use an immersion blender. Taste and adjust seasonings to your taste.

4. Serve immediately with a dollop of coconut yogurt and enjoy!

KETO BLUEBERRY MUFFINS

INGREDIENTS

- 1 cup almond flour
- 2 tsp baking powder
- 1/4 cup butter, melted
- 2 eggs
- 1/2 cup erythritol
- 1 cup blueberries

INSTRUCTIONS

1. Preheat your oven to 350 degrees.
2. In a medium bowl add almond flour, baking powder, eggs and erythritol. Mix well.

3. Melt butter and add to almond flour mixture.
4. Once fully combined, gently fold in blueberries. You can use fresh or frozen blueberries, but I feel like frozen blueberries tend to be consistent in their sweetness.
5. Pour batter into baking cups about halfway to the top. I love these baking cups and highly recommend them.
6. Bake for 25 minutes.

KETO CHOCOLATE PIE: EASY FRENCH SILK PIE

INGREDIENTS

Keto Chocolate Crust Ingredients

- 1½ cup almond flour
- 3 TBSP cocoa powder
- 1 egg
- 1/3 cup erythritol
- ¼ cup butter – not melted
- ½ tsp baking powder
- ¼ tsp salt
- 1 tsp vanilla extract

Keto Chocolate Pie Filling

- 16 oz cream cheese – set out at room temperature
- ¾ cup whipping cream
- 4 tbsp sour cream
- 3 oz dark chocolate – melted
- ½ cup unsweetened cocoa powder
- 1 tsp vanilla extract
- ½ cup erythritol

Keto Whipped Cream Topping

- 3/4 cup heavy cream
- 2 TBSP Swerve Powdered Sweetener
- 1 tsp vanilla extract

INSTRUCTIONS

How To Make A Keto Chocolate Pie Crust

1. Preheat oven to 375°F. Grease a 9-inch pie dish with cooking spray or butter.
2. In a large mixing bowl, add the almond flour, sweetener, cocoa powder, baking powder, salt, and cold butter. Mix well to

combine and be sure the butter is well incorporated.

3. Add the egg to the mixture and blend until the dough looks like crumbles.

4. Spread and flatten out the dough into the prepared pie dish. Bake for 15 minutes. Allow the pie crust to completely cool.

How To Make Keto Chocolate Filling

1. In a large mixing bowl, add cream cheese, whipped cream, sour cream, melted chocolate, cocoa powder, sweetener, and vanilla extract.

2. Blend for about 3-4 minutes or until the chocolate filling is light and fluffy.

3. Spread the chocolate filling into the baked pie crust and refrigerate for 4-6 hours.

How To Make Keto Whipped Cream Topping:

1. In a large bowl, use an electric hand mixer to blend the whipping cream, vanilla extract and powdered sweetener. Beat on high until peaks form.

2. Top the pie with whipped cream topping.

ANTI INFLAMMATORY GREEN JUICE

INGREDIENTS

- 2 cups fresh spinach, lightly packed (3 oz)
- 2 large cucumbers (1¼ lbs, peeled if not organic)
- 1 tsp fresh gingerroot (about ½ inch)
- ½ bunch flat-leaf parsley (2 oz)
- 2 large apples, cored (1 lb)
- ½ lemon, with peel (see notes)
- liquid stevia (optional, to taste)

INSTRUCTIONS

1. Wash and roughly chop all produce. Run through your juicer, alternating greens with juicy fruits and veggies.
2. Add a few drops of liquid stevia, if desired.

HEALING BREAKFAST PORRIDGE {INSTANT POT OPTION} – AIP OPTIONS

INGREDIENTS

- 2–3 tbsp lightly toasted sunflower seeds (or 1 Tbsp tahini)- if you can tolerate. For seed substitute, use an additional 2 tbsp of coconut flakes or coconut butter (grounded) See notes
- 2 tbsp unsweetened shredded coconut
- 1 tbsp chia seed or flaxseed (omit for AIP or substitute with 1 tbsp collagen/ gelatin powder)
- 1/2 tsp cinnamon
- 1 tsp ginger, ground
- pinch of turmeric, ground
- pinch of sea salt
- 1/2 cup water or coconut milk, more if needed
- 1 cup chopped squash, cooked (ex: butternut squash or kabocha/ or acorn squash).
- If using Instant pot you will need additional coconut oil or ghee and water

- pure maple syrup or raw honey

Extra toppings: berries or cherries, pomegranate seeds, coconut cream or coconut yogurt to top.

INSTRUCTIONS

Stove Top Instructions

1. Combine all dry ingredients (sunflower seeds, coconut chia, and spices and grind in a coffee grinder or blender until you get a flour-like consistency. If you are short on time, use tahini instead of sunflower seeds and just mix all together. SEE NOTES FOR SEEDLESS option.
2. .In a small bowl, add the dry mixture with water or coconut milk, let it adsorb and form a gel. Feel free to save a little bit of the gel for topping!
3. Scoop cooked squash and gel mixture into a blender and blend until smooth.
4. Heat the porridge stove-top on medium heat just until it starts to bubble. Stirring occasionally.

5. Remove from heat, pour into your favorite bowl, and top with the dry mixture you set aside.

1. 6. Optional Add in –>   1 tsp of ghee if desired, helps improve digestion and healthy fats help absorb the nutrients adding in more nourishment.

6. Top with fresh berries, extra milk, etc.

INSTANT POT OPTION

7. Peel and Chop your squash into large pieces. Place in the instant pot with 1 tbsp or less of coconut oil. Add in a pinch of cinnamon and nutmeg and sauté for 5 minutes, turning the squash.

8. Once the squash is coated, Add 1/3 cup of water to Pressure Cooker cooking pot and lock on lid, close pressure valve.

9. Cook on Manual High Pressure for 5-6 minutes.

10. Allow a 10 minute Natural Pressure Release. Or use a quick release if short on time. Release the lid, drain the water then puree the squash with a hand blender.

11. Mix in your other ingredients (dry mix and tahini/sesame mix) and a splash of milk (non dairy). Stir all together. Place the lid back on and keep it on warm mode until ready to serve. See notes for meal prep.

SALMON INSTANT POT RECIPE

INGREDIENTS

- 2 fresh or thawed salmon filets

- 1 large lemon cut into 4 slices

- 2 teaspoons dried dill

- 2 tablespoons extra virgin olive oil

- 1 cup water

INSTRUCTIONS

1. Fill bottom of Instant Pot with 1 cup of water.
2. Place 2 salmon filets on trivet inside Instant Pot.
3. Pour olive oil on top of filets.
4. Sprinkle dill seasoning over salmon filets.

5. Place 2 slices of lemon on each filet.
6. Shut Instant Pot and set to "sealing" function.
7. Select steam function and set for 3 minutes.
8. Quick release to release steam.
9. Plate salmon.

STRAWBERRY AND GREENS SMOOTHIE

INGREDIENTS

- 1 cup almond milk
- 1 frozen medium banana (or half large)
- 1/2 cup strawberries, fresh or frozen
- 1/2 cup spinach
- 1/2 cup kale
- 1 tbsp Udo's Oil 3-6-9 Blend
- sweetener of choice to taste, maple, agave, etc.

INSTRUCTIONS

1. Add the almond milk to the blender followed by the rest of the ingredients. If

using frozen strawberries add an additional
1/2 cup of water.
2. Blend until smooth and then taste and
   sweeten if desired.
3. Pour into a glass and enjoy!

TOMATO-LESS MARINARA SAUCE (NIGHTSHADE-FREE, AIP-FRIENDLY)

INGREDIENTS

- 1 tablespoon coconut oil
- 2 yellow onions , chopped
- 4 garlic cloves , minced
- 1 pound carrots , chopped
- 1 medium beet , chopped
- 1 cup water
- 1 teaspoon sea salt
- 2 tablespoons fresh lemon juice

INSTRUCTIONS

1. Melt the coconut oil in a large pot over
   medium heat, and saute the onions until they
   are tender and golden, about 10 minutes.

2. Add in the minced garlic and saute until
    fragrant, about 1 minute.
3. Add in the carrots, beet, and water and bring
    the mixture to a boil.
4.   Cover and lower the heat to a simmer,
    cooking until the carrots and beets are fork-
    tender, about 30 to 40 minutes.
5. Carefully transfer the mixture to a high-
    speed blender, add the salt and lemon juice,
    and blend until smooth. (Be sure to cover
    the vent in the lid of your blender with a
    dishtowel to prevent the top blowing off
    from the pressure of blending hot liquids!)
    Taste the sauce and adjust any seasonings,
    as needed, including a dash of oregano and
    basil, if you like! You can also add
    additional water, if you'd like a thinner
    sauce.
6. Serve warm over your favorite vegetable or
    pasta dish, and enjoy! Leftover sauce can be
    stored in a sealed container in the fridge for
    up to a week, or in the freezer for months.

GOLDEN MISO SOUP

INGREDIENTS

- 100 g / 3½ oz wholegrain noodles (I use whole wheat)
- 750 ml / 3 cups water
- ½ tsp vegetable bouillon powder (or ½ vegetable stock cube)
- 2 tsp ginger finely grated or minced
- ½ tsp ground turmeric
- ¼ tsp ground black pepper
- 100 g / 6 medium tenderstem broccoli stalks finely sliced
- 100 g / 5 medium chesnut mushrooms
- ½ sweet romano or red bell pepper finely diced
- 150 g / 5½ oz tofu drained and cubed* [See notes]
- ½ lime freshly squeezed
- 1½ TBSP white miso

INSTRUCTIONS

1. Prepare the noodles according to the instructions on the packet.

2. Meanwhile, bring 750ml water to a boil in a saucepan. Stir in the vegetable bouillon powder, ginger, turmeric and black pepper. Add the tenderstem broccoli, mushrooms, pepper and tofu, then reduce the heat to low. Stir in the lime juice and miso.

3. When the noodles are ready, add them to the broth to warm through. Divide the noodles between two bowls, ladle the broth and vegetables on top and serve.

4. The broth (without the noodles) can be stored in the fridge for up to three days. Gently heat through before serving.

CONCLUSION

The journey to a healthier life with lupus is a challenging one, but the rewards of eating a balanced, lupus-friendly diet can be great. With the right recipes and knowledge, you can be well on your way to improving your overall health and effectively managing your symptoms. The recipes in this cookbook are easy to follow and intended to help you on your journey to a healthier, more balanced lifestyle. With dedication and commitment to eating the right foods, you can be sure to experience an improved quality of life with lupus.

Good luck on your journey!